TRIBULUS TERRESTRIS:
A Comprehensive Guide

Boost Testosterone and Libido, Enhance Reproductive Wellness, Support Cardiovascular Health, Balance Hormones, and Promote Antioxidant and Anti-Inflammatory Benefits for Vitality

DR. KELLY O. MCNEILL

All rights reserved. No part of this book may be reproduced or transmitted in any form or by any means, electronic or mechanical, including photocopying, or by any information storage and retrieval system, without permission in writing from the publisher, except for brief quotations in critical reviews and certain other noncommercial uses permitted by copyright law.
© **Dr. Kelly O. McNeill, 2024.**

Table of Contents

Disclaimer vi
CHAPTER 1: 1
Introduction to Tribulus Terrestris 1
CHAPTER 2: 6
Understanding Testosterone and Libido . 6
CHAPTER 3: 14
Scientific Composition of Tribulus Terrestris 14
CHAPTER 4: 22
Health Benefits Beyond Testosterone 22
CHAPTER 5: 30
Tribulus Terrestris and Testosterone: Scientific Insights 30
CHAPTER 6: 39
Forms and Dosages of Tribulus Terrestris 39
CHAPTER 7: 50
Safety and Side Effects 50
CHAPTER 8: 60
Choosing High-Quality Tribulus Terrestris Supplements 60
CHAPTER 9: 71

Incorporating Tribulus Terrestris into Your Routine... 71

CHAPTER 10: 82

Conclusion and Future Perspectives 82

    Final Thoughts... 92

Disclaimer

The information provided in this book is for educational and informational purposes only and is not intended as medical advice. While every effort has been made to ensure the accuracy of the information, it is important to note that drug information is constantly evolving as new research and clinical practices emerge.

This book is not a substitute for professional medical advice, diagnosis, or treatment. Always seek the guidance of your physician, pharmacist, or other qualified healthcare provider with any questions you may have regarding a medical condition, medication, or treatment. Do not disregard professional medical advice or delay seeking it because of something you have read in this book.

The author and publisher are not responsible for any adverse effects, consequences, or damages resulting from the use of the information presented in this book. The medications discussed may have different effects on different individuals, and the dosages or treatments mentioned may not be suitable for everyone. The mention of specific drugs, dosages, or treatment options is not an endorsement or recommendation.

For personalized medical advice, consult with a licensed healthcare provider before starting, changing, or discontinuing any medication or treatment plan.

CHAPTER 1:
Introduction to Tribulus Terrestris

Overview of the Plant

Tribulus Terrestris, often referred to as "puncture vine," is a small, flowering plant that thrives in harsh, dry environments. Recognizable by its spiny fruit and delicate yellow flowers, this hardy plant is far more than just a resilient weed. It belongs to the Zygophyllaceae family and is often celebrated in traditional medicine for its potential health benefits.

The plant's appeal lies in its bioactive compounds, particularly saponins, which are believed to contribute to its effects on human health. While modern science is still unraveling its full range of benefits, Tribulus Terrestris has long been a staple in natural remedies for boosting vitality and improving overall wellness.

History and Traditional Uses

Tribulus Terrestris has a rich history, with its use tracing back thousands of years in various cultures. In traditional Chinese medicine, it was regarded as a remedy for liver and kidney health, as well as an aphrodisiac. Similarly, in Ayurveda—the ancient healing system of India—it was known as *Gokshura* and used to support urinary and reproductive health. Practitioners praised its ability to balance bodily functions and enhance stamina.

In ancient Greece, the plant was used to boost energy and combat fatigue. By the Middle Ages, its reputation as a sexual tonic and physical enhancer had spread across Europe and the Middle East. In African traditional medicine, Tribulus was often employed as a diuretic and an anti-inflammatory agent.

The enduring appeal of Tribulus lies in its dual reputation as both a therapeutic herb and a performance enhancer. This balance of traditional wisdom and anecdotal success stories has kept the plant in the spotlight for centuries.

Geographical Distribution

Tribulus Terrestris is a global traveler, flourishing in a wide range of climates and terrains. Native to southern Europe, Asia, Africa, and Australia, it thrives in regions with arid or semi-arid conditions. It is particularly resilient, capable of growing in poor soils and surviving extreme drought.

Today, the plant is found on nearly every continent, from the sandy plains of India to the rugged deserts of the southwestern United States. Its adaptability has made it a common sight in disturbed areas, such as roadsides, fields, and even urban landscapes.

Despite its unassuming appearance, Tribulus Terrestris has made a significant impact on both traditional medicine and modern herbal supplementation. Its widespread availability ensures that this ancient plant continues to play a vital role in wellness practices around the world.

A Plant That Bridges Past and Present

Tribulus Terrestris is more than just a herb; it is a testament to the enduring connection between humanity and nature. By understanding its roots—both literal and historical—we can better appreciate the potential this plant holds for modern health. From its use in ancient remedies to its growing popularity in the wellness industry,

Tribulus Terrestris remains a fascinating subject for exploration.

In this chapter, we've begun to uncover the layers of history, geography, and cultural significance surrounding this humble yet powerful plant. As we progress through this guidebook, we will delve deeper into the science and practical applications that make Tribulus a noteworthy addition to any health-conscious individual's routine.

CHAPTER 2:

Understanding Testosterone and Libido

Testosterone and libido are deeply interconnected elements of human biology, impacting not just our physical health but also our emotional well-being. While these terms are often discussed in the context of men's health, they are relevant to all genders, albeit in different capacities. Let's unravel the fascinating interplay between testosterone and libido, exploring their biological roles, the factors influencing sexual desire, and the common hurdles posed by hormonal imbalances.

Biological Roles of Testosterone

Testosterone is often labeled the "male hormone," but this oversimplifies its critical functions. Produced primarily in the testes in men and in smaller amounts by the ovaries and adrenal glands in women, testosterone plays a vital role in various physiological processes:

- **Sexual Development and Reproductive Health**: Testosterone is essential for the development of male reproductive organs during puberty. It also drives sperm production and supports libido in men. In women, it contributes to sexual arousal and overall energy levels.
- **Muscle Growth and Bone Density**: This hormone promotes muscle protein synthesis, leading to muscle growth and improved strength. It also supports

bone density, reducing the risk of fractures as we age.

- **Mood Regulation and Cognitive Function**:
Testosterone affects brain chemistry, contributing to mood stabilization, motivation, and cognitive sharpness. Imbalances can lead to mood swings, irritability, and even depression.

- **Energy Levels and Overall Vitality**:
Testosterone fuels physical energy, endurance, and a general sense of vitality. Low levels can leave individuals feeling fatigued and unmotivated.

While testosterone levels naturally decline with age, lifestyle choices and health conditions can significantly influence these levels.

Factors Influencing Libido

Libido, or sexual desire, is a complex interplay of physical, psychological, and social factors. It is neither static nor uniform, varying widely from person to person and even across different phases of an individual's life.

- **Hormonal Influence:** Testosterone is a primary driver of libido in both men and women. When levels drop due to aging, stress, or medical conditions, a corresponding decline in sexual desire is often observed.
- **Emotional and Psychological Health:** Anxiety, depression, and low self-esteem can dampen libido. Relationship dynamics, such as unresolved conflicts or lack of emotional intimacy, also play a significant role.

- **Lifestyle Factors**: Poor diet, lack of exercise, and insufficient sleep can negatively impact libido. Excessive alcohol consumption and smoking further exacerbate the issue by impairing hormonal balance and blood flow.
- **Cultural and Social Context**: Societal norms, stress from work or family responsibilities, and even exposure to unrealistic portrayals of sexuality in media can shape one's libido, sometimes causing it to decline due to pressure or unmet expectations.

Common Issues with Hormonal Imbalances

Hormonal imbalances are among the most common reasons for disruptions in testosterone levels and libido. These imbalances can stem from a variety of causes:

- **Low Testosterone (Hypogonadism):**
In men, hypogonadism can lead to fatigue, reduced muscle mass, erectile dysfunction, and decreased libido. In women, low testosterone is linked to diminished sexual desire and energy.
- **Hyperprolactinemia:**
Elevated prolactin levels, often caused by pituitary gland issues, can suppress testosterone production, reducing libido.
- **Thyroid Disorders:**
Both hypothyroidism and hyperthyroidism can interfere with sex hormone production, affecting desire and performance.
- **Polycystic Ovary Syndrome (PCOS):**
In women, PCOS is a condition where hormonal imbalances can lead to

irregular testosterone levels, impacting libido and overall health.

- **Stress and Cortisol Levels**: Chronic stress elevates cortisol, a hormone that suppresses testosterone production, leading to diminished libido and energy levels.
- **Medications and Medical Conditions**: Certain medications, such as antidepressants and blood pressure drugs, can interfere with testosterone and libido. Additionally, conditions like diabetes and obesity are closely linked to hormonal imbalances that affect sexual health.

Bridging Knowledge to Action

Understanding the roles of testosterone and libido, along with the factors that influence them, is the first step in taking proactive measures. A healthy lifestyle, regular medical checkups, and open communication about sexual health are crucial for maintaining a balanced and fulfilling life.

Tribulus Terrestris, the focus of this guide, may offer a natural means of addressing some of these challenges by potentially supporting healthy testosterone levels and enhancing libido. As we move forward, we'll explore how this remarkable plant fits into the broader context of hormonal health and vitality.

CHAPTER 3:

Scientific Composition of Tribulus Terrestris

Tribulus Terrestris, often hailed as a natural remedy for boosting vitality, owes its reputation to its unique scientific composition. Beneath its humble, spiny exterior lies a treasure trove of bioactive compounds that interact with the human body in fascinating ways. In this chapter, we delve into the plant's key chemical constituents, the mechanisms through which it exerts its effects, and its overall nutritional profile.

Key Bioactive Compounds

Tribulus Terrestris is rich in a variety of phytochemicals that are responsible for its therapeutic properties. These include:

- **Saponins**:
  The most well-studied compounds in Tribulus Terrestris are steroidal saponins, particularly *protodioscin*. These saponins are believed to mimic the effects of certain hormones, making them a key factor in the plant's reputation for enhancing libido and testosterone.
- **Flavonoids**:
  Flavonoids in Tribulus act as antioxidants, combating oxidative stress and reducing inflammation in the body. This contributes to overall health and may support recovery after physical exertion.

- **Alkaloids**:
  Alkaloids present in the plant exhibit a variety of bioactivities, including antimicrobial and anti-inflammatory effects.
- **Glycosides**:
  Glycosides in Tribulus Terrestris are thought to contribute to its diuretic and tonic properties, supporting urinary and kidney health.
- **Phytosterols**:
  These plant-based compounds help in lowering cholesterol levels and may contribute to heart health.

Mechanisms of Action

Tribulus Terrestris operates through several biological pathways, making it a versatile supplement with multiple health benefits.

1. **Hormonal Modulation**:
   The saponins in Tribulus, particularly

protodioscin, are thought to stimulate the production of luteinizing hormone (LH) in the body. LH, in turn, signals the testes in men and ovaries in women to produce testosterone and other sex hormones. This action may explain its reputation as a testosterone booster and libido enhancer.

2. **Nitric Oxide Production**: Tribulus has been shown to enhance the production of nitric oxide, a molecule that improves blood flow by dilating blood vessels. This effect not only supports cardiovascular health but also plays a role in improving erectile function.

3. **Antioxidant Activity**: The flavonoids and other antioxidant compounds in Tribulus neutralize harmful free radicals, reducing oxidative stress. This contributes to its

protective effects on various organs, including the liver and kidneys.

4. **Anti-Inflammatory Effects**: Tribulus may suppress inflammatory pathways, aiding in the management of conditions like arthritis and promoting faster recovery from exercise-induced muscle damage.

5. **Diuretic Action**: Traditionally used as a diuretic, Tribulus supports urinary health by promoting the excretion of excess fluids and toxins, which can help prevent kidney stones and urinary tract infections.

6. **Antimicrobial Properties**: Some studies suggest that Tribulus exhibits antibacterial and antifungal properties, making it a potential aid in managing infections.

Nutritional Profile

Beyond its bioactive compounds, Tribulus Terrestris also offers a modest but noteworthy nutritional profile:

- **Vitamins**:
  The plant contains small amounts of vitamins such as vitamin C, which supports immunity, and B-complex vitamins, essential for energy production and nervous system health.
- **Minerals**:
  Tribulus is a source of essential minerals like potassium, magnesium, and zinc. Potassium and magnesium are crucial for maintaining electrolyte balance and muscle function, while zinc is known to support immune health and testosterone production.
- **Carbohydrates and Fiber**:
  The plant provides carbohydrates for

energy and dietary fiber, which aids digestion and promotes gut health.

- **Proteins and Amino Acids**: Although not a significant source of protein, Tribulus contains small amounts of amino acids that contribute to its overall nutritional benefits.

Synergy of Compounds

What makes Tribulus Terrestris particularly effective is the synergy among its various compounds. For example, the saponins work alongside flavonoids and alkaloids to deliver comprehensive benefits, from hormonal balance to improved circulation and antioxidant protection. This natural synergy is a hallmark of herbal medicine, where the whole plant often outperforms isolated extracts.

Balancing Nature and Science

Tribulus Terrestris sits at the crossroads of traditional wisdom and modern scientific inquiry. While its bioactive compounds and mechanisms of action are well-documented, ongoing research continues to shed light on how this remarkable plant can be harnessed for optimal health.

As we explore further chapters, we will discuss how these scientific insights translate into practical applications, from supplement formulation to everyday health routines. By understanding the intricate composition of Tribulus Terrestris, we gain a deeper appreciation for its potential to enhance well-being in a holistic and natural way.

CHAPTER 4:
Health Benefits Beyond Testosterone

Tribulus Terrestris is often celebrated for its role in enhancing testosterone levels and libido, but its benefits extend far beyond hormonal health. This versatile herb has been a cornerstone of traditional medicine for centuries, with emerging scientific research validating its potential in various areas, including cardiovascular health, urinary and reproductive wellness, and as a source of powerful antioxidant and anti-inflammatory properties.

Effects on Cardiovascular Health

The heart is the engine of life, and maintaining its health is crucial for overall well-being. Tribulus Terrestris may offer several cardiovascular benefits, primarily through its ability to improve blood flow and manage lipid levels.

- **Blood Pressure Regulation**: Tribulus has shown promise in lowering blood pressure by promoting the production of nitric oxide. This compound helps relax and widen blood vessels, improving circulation and reducing strain on the heart. This vasodilation effect may also explain its traditional use in managing heart-related conditions.
- **Cholesterol Management**: Studies suggest that Tribulus Terrestris can help regulate cholesterol levels by reducing LDL (bad cholesterol) and increasing HDL (good cholesterol). This balance is vital for preventing the

buildup of arterial plaques, a key contributor to heart disease.

- **Enhanced Blood Flow**: The plant's impact on nitric oxide levels also supports better blood flow throughout the body. This not only benefits cardiovascular health but can also improve energy levels, stamina, and recovery after physical exertion.

While more research is needed to fully understand the scope of its cardiovascular benefits, the initial findings are promising, particularly for individuals looking to support heart health naturally.

Role in Managing Urinary and Reproductive Health

Tribulus Terrestris has long been used in traditional medicine to address issues related to the urinary and reproductive systems.

Modern research is beginning to catch up, shedding light on its potential in these areas.

- **Urinary Health**: Known for its diuretic properties, Tribulus encourages the elimination of excess water and toxins from the body. This action helps prevent the formation of kidney stones and supports the treatment of urinary tract infections (UTIs). Additionally, its anti-inflammatory effects may ease symptoms associated with bladder discomfort and irritation.
- **Reproductive Health**: In men, Tribulus is often used to support sperm quality and motility, which are critical factors in fertility. Its potential to boost testosterone levels indirectly contributes to improved reproductive function.

For women, Tribulus has been explored as a natural remedy for menstrual irregularities and hormonal imbalances. Some studies suggest it may alleviate symptoms of polycystic ovary syndrome (PCOS) by helping regulate hormone levels and improve ovarian function.

- **Sexual Wellness**: Beyond its testosterone-boosting effects, Tribulus is believed to enhance overall sexual satisfaction by improving blood flow to reproductive organs and reducing stress-related barriers to intimacy.

Antioxidant and Anti-inflammatory Properties

Oxidative stress and inflammation are two major contributors to chronic diseases, from arthritis to cardiovascular issues. Tribulus

Terrestris is rich in compounds that combat these harmful processes, making it a powerful ally in promoting long-term health.

- **Antioxidant Effects**: Tribulus contains flavonoids and other phytochemicals that neutralize free radicals—unstable molecules that can damage cells and accelerate aging. By reducing oxidative stress, these antioxidants protect vital organs, including the heart, liver, and kidneys.
- **Anti-inflammatory Action**: Inflammation is the body's natural response to injury or infection, but chronic inflammation can lead to diseases such as diabetes, arthritis, and even cancer. Tribulus helps regulate inflammatory pathways, reducing excessive inflammation without compromising the body's ability to heal.

- **Liver and Kidney Protection**: Research indicates that Tribulus may shield the liver and kidneys from damage caused by toxins or oxidative stress. This protective effect is particularly beneficial for individuals exposed to environmental pollutants or those taking medications that strain these organs.
- **Support for Joint Health**: The plant's anti-inflammatory properties may also extend to joint health, offering relief for individuals with conditions like arthritis or general joint pain from overuse or aging.

A Holistic Wellness Ally

While Tribulus Terrestris is often marketed for its effects on testosterone, its broader health benefits cannot be overlooked. Its ability to support cardiovascular health, enhance urinary and reproductive function, and provide antioxidant and anti-inflammatory protection makes it a versatile herb for anyone seeking a holistic approach to wellness.

As we move through this guide, we will continue to explore how Tribulus can be integrated into daily life to maximize its diverse health benefits. Whether you're looking to address specific concerns or simply enhance your overall vitality, this remarkable plant has much to offer beyond its reputation as a testosterone booster.

CHAPTER 5:

Tribulus Terrestris and Testosterone: Scientific Insights

Tribulus Terrestris has become synonymous with testosterone enhancement and libido improvement, making it a staple in many supplements marketed for men's health. But how much of this reputation is backed by science, and where does speculation take over? In this chapter, we'll dive into the research on Tribulus Terrestris, examining its testosterone-boosting effects, libido-enhancing properties, and the controversies and limitations surrounding these claims.

Research on Testosterone-Boosting Effects

Tribulus Terrestris first gained popularity as a natural testosterone booster after Eastern European athletes reportedly used it in the 1980s to enhance performance. Modern research, however, has revealed a mixed picture.

- **Positive Findings**: Some studies suggest that the saponins in Tribulus, particularly protodioscin, may stimulate the release of luteinizing hormone (LH), which signals the testes to produce testosterone. This mechanism has been observed in animal studies, where Tribulus supplementation led to increased testosterone levels, enhanced sperm production, and improved reproductive health.

For example, a study conducted on rats found that Tribulus significantly raised testosterone levels and improved sexual performance. This supports the idea that the plant may have a role in hormonal regulation under certain conditions.

- **Inconclusive Human Studies**: While the evidence in animals is promising, human studies are less consistent. Some trials show that Tribulus supplementation can improve testosterone levels in men with low baseline testosterone, especially when combined with a healthy lifestyle. However, other studies indicate no significant change in testosterone levels among healthy men or athletes using Tribulus.

One double-blind, placebo-controlled study conducted on athletes found no measurable increase in testosterone levels after several weeks of Tribulus supplementation. This highlights the importance of context, as the plant's effects may depend on the individual's hormonal baseline or other physiological factors.

Studies on Libido Enhancement

While the connection between Tribulus and testosterone remains debated, its reputation as a libido enhancer is more robust. Multiple studies have highlighted its potential to improve sexual desire and satisfaction in both men and women.

- **Mechanisms of Action**: Tribulus is believed to increase nitric oxide levels, which enhances blood flow to the sexual organs. This improved circulation can positively affect erectile function in men and sensitivity in women, contributing to heightened arousal and pleasure.

- **Research in Men**: A study published in the *Journal of Sexual Medicine* demonstrated that Tribulus significantly improved erectile function, libido, and satisfaction in men experiencing mild to moderate erectile dysfunction. Importantly, these benefits were observed even in the absence of significant testosterone changes, suggesting that Tribulus may work through mechanisms independent of hormonal modulation.
- **Research in Women**: Tribulus is not exclusively a male tonic. In a study on women with low libido, Tribulus supplementation was found to improve sexual desire, arousal, and satisfaction. Researchers attributed these effects to the plant's potential role

in balancing sex hormones and enhancing blood flow.

These findings make Tribulus a valuable natural option for individuals seeking to enhance their sexual wellness without resorting to pharmaceutical solutions.

Controversies and Limitations

Despite its popularity, Tribulus Terrestris remains a topic of debate in the scientific community.

- **Inconsistent Results**: One of the main controversies lies in the variability of study outcomes. While some trials highlight Tribulus's positive effects on testosterone and libido, others fail to find significant benefits. Factors such as study design, dosage, and the quality of the Tribulus extract used may contribute to these inconsistencies.

- **Placebo Effect**: Sexual desire and performance are heavily influenced by psychological factors. Some researchers argue that Tribulus's libido-enhancing effects may partly stem from the placebo effect, where individuals experience improvement because they believe in the supplement's efficacy.
- **Exaggerated Marketing Claims**: The supplement industry often markets Tribulus as a miracle testosterone booster, which can create unrealistic expectations. This oversimplification neglects the nuanced role that Tribulus plays in hormonal and sexual health.
- **Lack of Standardization**: Not all Tribulus supplements are created equal. Variability in saponin content, extraction methods, and

quality control can significantly impact a product's effectiveness. Consumers should look for reputable brands that standardize their extracts for saponin content, particularly protodioscin.

- **Population-Specific Effects**: Tribulus may be more effective in individuals with specific conditions, such as hypogonadism (low testosterone) or sexual dysfunction. For healthy individuals with normal testosterone levels, the benefits may be less pronounced.

Balancing Expectations with Evidence

Tribulus Terrestris occupies an intriguing space in the world of herbal medicine. While it's not a guaranteed solution for boosting testosterone, the existing research supports its potential to improve sexual health and quality of life, especially in individuals with underlying hormonal imbalances or sexual dysfunction.

As with any supplement, it's essential to approach Tribulus with informed expectations. While it may not transform everyone into a superhuman athlete, its centuries-old reputation as a vitality booster and modern scientific insights suggest it can be a valuable part of a holistic wellness regimen.

The next chapters will explore how to incorporate Tribulus effectively into your routine and combine it with other lifestyle strategies to maximize its benefits. Understanding both the promise and the limitations of this remarkable plant is key to harnessing its full potential.

CHAPTER 6:

Forms and Dosages of Tribulus Terrestris

Tribulus Terrestris is available in a variety of forms, each offering unique benefits depending on the needs and preferences of the individual. While this natural supplement is celebrated for its wide-ranging health benefits, achieving optimal results requires an understanding of the different formulations, proper dosing, and the potential risks associated with overuse. In this chapter, we'll explore the commonly available forms of Tribulus, recommended dosages for various purposes, and the precautions needed to use it safely and effectively.

Forms of Tribulus Terrestris

Tribulus Terrestris is processed into several forms to make it convenient for consumption. Each form has its advantages, depending on lifestyle and health goals.

1. **Capsules and Tablets**:
     - **Overview**: Capsules and tablets are the most popular form of Tribulus supplementation. They are convenient, easy to dose, and often standardized to contain a specific percentage of saponins, the plant's primary active compounds.
     - **Ideal for**: Individuals who prefer simplicity and precise dosing. Capsules and tablets are also the most travel-friendly option.
2. **Powders**:

- **Overview**: Tribulus powder is made by grinding dried plant material, usually the fruit or aerial parts. Powders can be mixed into smoothies, teas, or other beverages.
- **Ideal for**: Those who enjoy customizing their intake or prefer natural, less-processed supplements. Powders are also cost-effective for long-term use.

3. **Liquid Extracts and Tinctures**:
    - **Overview**: Liquid forms are created by steeping the plant material in alcohol or glycerin to extract its active compounds. These are highly concentrated and absorbed quickly by the body.
    - **Ideal for**: People who need rapid absorption or prefer to avoid swallowing pills. Tinctures

also allow for easy dose adjustments.
4. **Teas and Infusions**:
    - **Overview**: Traditional use of Tribulus often involves brewing it into a tea. This method is less potent but aligns with the traditional practices of herbal medicine.
    - **Ideal for**: Individuals seeking a gentle, soothing way to enjoy Tribulus, often as part of a holistic wellness routine.

Recommended Dosages Based on Purpose

The dosage of Tribulus Terrestris can vary depending on the form of the supplement, its concentration, and the desired outcome. While there's no universal dosage, research and traditional practices provide guidelines to follow:

1. **For General Health and Vitality**:
   - Dosage: 250–750 mg of a standardized extract (containing 40–60% saponins) daily.
   - Purpose: Supports overall energy levels, reduces oxidative stress, and promotes hormonal balance.
2. **For Testosterone and Libido Enhancement**:
   - Dosage: 750–1,500 mg of standardized extract daily.
   - Purpose: Stimulates hormone production and enhances sexual function. Effects may take a few weeks to become noticeable.
3. **For Athletic Performance and Recovery**:

- Dosage: 1,000–2,000 mg of standardized extract daily, often divided into two doses.
- Purpose: Enhances stamina, supports muscle recovery, and reduces exercise-induced oxidative stress.

4. **For Urinary and Reproductive Health**:
    - Dosage: 500–1,000 mg of standardized extract daily.
    - Purpose: Addresses mild urinary tract issues, supports fertility, and improves reproductive health.

Risks of Overdosage

Like any supplement, Tribulus Terrestris should be used responsibly to avoid adverse effects. While it is generally considered safe, excessive consumption can lead to potential risks.

1. **Common Side Effects**:
   - Nausea, stomach upset, or diarrhea may occur, especially when taken on an empty stomach or in high doses.
   - Mild allergic reactions, such as skin rash or itching, have been reported in sensitive individuals.
2. **Hormonal Imbalance**:
   - Excessive intake of Tribulus may disrupt hormonal balance, leading to unintended effects such as mood swings, excessive hair growth, or acne in susceptible individuals.
3. **Impact on Kidney and Liver Function**:
   - Prolonged high doses may strain the liver or kidneys, especially in

individuals with pre-existing conditions. Although rare, overuse can increase the risk of toxicity.

4. **Interference with Medications**:
   - Tribulus may interact with certain medications, such as hormone replacement therapies, diuretics, or blood pressure drugs. Always consult a healthcare provider before starting supplementation, especially if you are on medication.

5. **Safety for Specific Populations**:
   - Pregnant or breastfeeding women should avoid Tribulus due to its potential effects on hormone levels.
   - Individuals with hormone-sensitive conditions, such as prostate cancer or PCOS, should

use Tribulus only under medical supervision.

How to Use Tribulus Safely

To minimize risks and maximize benefits, follow these guidelines when using Tribulus Terrestris:

- **Start Low and Adjust**: Begin with the lowest recommended dose and gradually increase as needed. This helps the body adapt and minimizes potential side effects.
- **Choose Standardized Extracts**: Look for products that specify the percentage of saponins, ensuring consistent potency and efficacy.
- **Cycle Your Usage**: Avoid taking Tribulus continuously for extended periods. A common approach is cycling,

such as taking it for six weeks followed by a two-week break.
- **Combine with a Healthy Lifestyle**: Supplements work best when combined with a balanced diet, regular exercise, and adequate sleep.
- **Monitor for Side Effects**: Pay attention to how your body responds, and discontinue use if you experience adverse effects.

Tribulus Terrestris is a versatile herb that can be tailored to meet various health goals, from enhancing vitality to supporting hormonal balance. By understanding the available forms, recommended dosages, and potential risks, you can make informed decisions about incorporating this powerful plant into your wellness routine. Always prioritize safety, quality, and moderation to unlock the full potential of Tribulus while safeguarding your health.

CHAPTER 7:

Safety and Side Effects

Tribulus Terrestris, though widely regarded as a natural and effective herbal remedy, is not without its safety considerations. Like any supplement, its use requires a thorough understanding of potential side effects, interactions with medications, and specific precautions for certain populations. This chapter aims to provide a balanced view of the safety profile of Tribulus, enabling users to make informed decisions about its inclusion in their health regimen.

Potential Side Effects and Contraindications

Tribulus Terrestris is generally considered safe when taken in appropriate doses, but excessive use or individual sensitivities can lead to adverse effects.

1. **Common Side Effects**:
    - **Digestive Issues**: Some individuals may experience mild gastrointestinal discomfort, including nausea, diarrhea, or stomach cramps, particularly when Tribulus is taken on an empty stomach or in high doses.
    - **Allergic Reactions**: While rare, some users report allergic responses such as itching, rashes, or hives. These symptoms warrant immediate discontinuation and medical consultation.
    - **Hormonal Effects**: Tribulus can influence hormone levels, which may lead to side effects like acne, mood swings, or

irregular menstrual cycles in sensitive individuals.

2. **Severe Side Effects (Rare)**:
   - Tribulus may cause a significant drop in blood sugar levels, posing a risk for individuals with diabetes or those prone to hypoglycemia.
   - Excessive use can potentially strain the kidneys or liver, particularly in individuals with pre-existing conditions affecting these organs.

3. **Contraindications**:
   - Pregnant and breastfeeding women should avoid Tribulus due to its potential to influence hormonal activity, which could harm fetal development or affect lactation.
   - Individuals with hormone-sensitive conditions, such as

breast cancer, prostate cancer, or endometriosis, should use Tribulus cautiously or avoid it altogether.

Interactions with Medications

Tribulus Terrestris has bioactive compounds that may interact with certain medications, either enhancing or diminishing their effects.

1. **Hormonal Medications**:
    - Tribulus may interfere with hormone replacement therapies or contraceptives by altering the body's natural hormonal balance. This can lead to reduced efficacy of these treatments.
2. **Blood Sugar Medications**:
    - Tribulus's potential to lower blood sugar levels may amplify the effects of antidiabetic drugs,

increasing the risk of hypoglycemia. Individuals managing diabetes should consult their healthcare provider before use.

3. **Diuretics**:
    - Known for its mild diuretic properties, Tribulus can interact with diuretic medications, potentially leading to excessive fluid loss or electrolyte imbalances.

4. **Blood Pressure Medications**:
    - Tribulus's ability to relax blood vessels and lower blood pressure may enhance the effects of antihypertensive drugs, increasing the risk of hypotension.

5. **Anticoagulants and Antiplatelets**:
    - Tribulus may have a mild blood-thinning effect, which could

interact with medications like aspirin, warfarin, or clopidogrel, increasing the risk of bleeding.

Precautions for Specific Populations

While Tribulus Terrestris offers numerous benefits, certain groups should approach its use with extra caution or avoid it altogether.

1. **Pregnant and Breastfeeding Women**:
    - The herb's potential to influence hormones makes it unsuitable for use during pregnancy, as it could potentially stimulate uterine contractions or affect hormonal balance. Similarly, its effects on breast milk production are not well-studied, so it is best avoided during breastfeeding.

2. **Individuals with Hormone-Sensitive Conditions**:
   - Tribulus's potential to modulate hormone levels could exacerbate conditions such as prostate cancer, breast cancer, or uterine fibroids. Consultation with a healthcare provider is essential before use in these cases.
3. **People with Chronic Illnesses**:
   - Individuals with chronic liver or kidney conditions should be cautious, as high doses of Tribulus might strain these organs. Regular monitoring of liver and kidney function is advisable for long-term users.
4. **Diabetic Individuals**:
   - Tribulus's blood sugar-lowering effects can be both a benefit and a risk. Diabetic individuals should carefully monitor their

blood sugar levels and adjust their medications under medical supervision.

5. **Athletes**:
    o While Tribulus is popular among athletes for its potential to boost performance, users should be aware of quality standards. Substandard supplements may be contaminated with banned substances, leading to issues during doping tests.

Practical Tips for Safe Use

To enjoy the benefits of Tribulus Terrestris while minimizing risks, consider the following guidelines:

- **Start with Low Doses**: Begin with the lowest recommended dose and gradually increase it based on tolerance and effectiveness.

- **Choose Reputable Brands**: Look for supplements that are third-party tested for purity and standardized for saponin content. Avoid unverified products that may contain harmful additives.
- **Consult a Healthcare Provider**: Always discuss Tribulus use with a healthcare professional, especially if you have pre-existing medical conditions, are on medication, or belong to a high-risk population.
- **Monitor for Side Effects**: Pay close attention to how your body reacts, and discontinue use if you experience adverse effects.
- **Follow Recommended Dosages**: Avoid exceeding the suggested daily intake, as higher doses do not necessarily translate to better results and may increase the risk of side effects.

Tribulus Terrestris is a powerful herbal supplement with a range of potential health benefits, but it is not without its risks. By understanding its side effects, interactions, and precautions, users can make informed decisions about its use. When taken responsibly, Tribulus can be a safe and effective addition to a holistic health regimen, helping individuals unlock its full potential while safeguarding their well-being.

CHAPTER 8:

Choosing High-Quality Tribulus Terrestris Supplements

As the popularity of Tribulus Terrestris grows, so does the variety of supplements available on the market. While this offers consumers many options, it also introduces the challenge of finding high-quality, authentic products. Unfortunately, not all supplements are created equal, and choosing a low-quality or adulterated product can compromise safety and effectiveness. In this chapter, we'll explore practical tips for identifying authentic Tribulus Terrestris products, understanding quality certifications, and avoiding adulterated or ineffective supplements.

How to Identify Authentic Products

Navigating the world of supplements can feel overwhelming, but knowing what to look for can make all the difference. Authentic Tribulus Terrestris supplements share certain key characteristics:

1. **Standardized Extracts**:
    - Look for products that specify the percentage of active compounds, such as **saponins** (typically 40–60%). Standardized extracts ensure consistent potency and effectiveness.
    - Avoid supplements that only list "Tribulus Terrestris" without detailing the concentration of active ingredients, as they may contain ineffective doses.
2. **Source of the Plant**:

- High-quality supplements often indicate the geographical origin of the plant. Tribulus grown in regions like **India**, **Bulgaria**, or **China** is widely regarded for its potency.
- Bulgarian Tribulus, in particular, is renowned for its high levels of protodioscin, a saponin linked to testosterone and libido enhancement.

3. **Transparent Ingredient Lists**:
   - Authentic products will have a clear, detailed label listing all ingredients, including the type of extract (fruit, leaf, or whole plant).
   - Avoid products with vague or incomplete ingredient lists, as they may contain fillers, additives, or undisclosed substances.

4. **Reputable Brands**:
    o Choose supplements from well-known, trusted brands with a proven track record of quality. Established companies often invest in rigorous testing and adhere to industry standards.
    o Research the brand online and read customer reviews to gauge product efficacy and company reliability.

Recognizing Quality Certifications

Quality certifications serve as a hallmark of trust, indicating that a supplement has undergone stringent testing and meets established standards. When shopping for Tribulus Terrestris, keep an eye out for the following certifications:

1. **Good Manufacturing Practices (GMP)**:
   - Supplements labeled with "GMP Certified" have been manufactured under strict quality control guidelines to ensure safety, purity, and potency.
   - This certification is a must-have for any supplement you consider.
2. **Third-Party Testing**:
   - Look for supplements that have been tested by independent laboratories to verify ingredient accuracy and the absence of contaminants like heavy metals or pesticides.
   - Labels such as **NSF Certified**, **USP Verified**, or **Informed-Choice** indicate thorough third-party testing.
3. **Organic Certification**:

- For those concerned about pesticides or synthetic chemicals, choose supplements labeled as **USDA Organic** or certified by similar organizations in your region.
- Organic certifications ensure that the product has been sourced and processed without harmful chemicals.

4. **Non-GMO Verified**:
    - Supplements bearing the **Non-GMO Project Verified** label guarantee that the product is free from genetically modified organisms, appealing to those seeking natural solutions.

5. **ISO Certification**:
    - International Organization for Standardization (ISO) certifications indicate that the manufacturing processes meet

global standards for safety and quality.

Avoiding Adulterated Supplements

Adulteration is a significant concern in the supplement industry, with some products containing undisclosed or harmful ingredients. These can pose serious health risks and diminish the credibility of Tribulus Terrestris. To avoid such pitfalls, follow these tips:

1. **Be Skeptical of Over-the-Top Claims**:
    - Products promising "instant results," "miraculous testosterone boosts," or "cures for all ailments" are likely too good to be true. Legitimate supplements offer gradual benefits, not quick fixes.

2. **Avoid Proprietary Blends**:
    - Some supplements list "proprietary blends" on their labels, which can obscure the actual amounts of active ingredients. These blends may include ineffective doses or unnecessary fillers.
3. **Steer Clear of Unverified Online Sellers**:
    - Stick to reputable online retailers or the brand's official website. Counterfeit or adulterated supplements are often sold through unverified third-party vendors.
    - Check for a money-back guarantee or return policy as an added layer of assurance.
4. **Inspect Packaging and Labels**:
    - Poor-quality packaging, misspelled words, or unclear

branding can signal a fake product. Legitimate supplements come in professionally designed packaging with clear instructions and contact information for the manufacturer.

5. **Request Certificates of Analysis (COA):**
    - Reputable brands will provide a Certificate of Analysis upon request. This document confirms that the product has been tested for purity and potency.

Practical Steps to Ensure Quality

When purchasing Tribulus Terrestris supplements, consider these additional steps to make an informed decision:

1. **Research Before Buying:**

- Spend time researching the product, brand, and reviews from verified buyers. Pay attention to any recurring complaints about effectiveness or side effects.

2. **Consult Healthcare Professionals**:
   - Before starting any supplement, discuss it with your doctor or a qualified nutritionist. They can provide personalized advice based on your health needs and existing medications.

3. **Choose Trusted Retailers**:
   - Purchase from established health stores, pharmacies, or credible online platforms like Amazon (ensuring the product is sold by the brand or an authorized distributor).

4. **Evaluate Price vs. Quality**:

- While affordability is important, avoid extremely cheap supplements, as they may compromise quality. High-quality Tribulus supplements often come at a reasonable premium due to rigorous sourcing and testing.

Tribulus Terrestris supplements can be a valuable addition to your wellness routine, but quality matters. By understanding how to identify authentic products, recognizing trusted certifications, and avoiding adulterated supplements, you can confidently choose a product that meets your health needs. Taking the time to verify your supplement ensures not only better results but also your safety and peace of mind. Always remember: informed choices lead to empowered health.

CHAPTER 9:

Incorporating Tribulus Terrestris into Your Routine

Adding Tribulus Terrestris to your health regimen can be an effective way to enhance well-being, whether you're seeking to boost testosterone, improve libido, or support overall vitality. However, to maximize its benefits, it's essential to integrate it thoughtfully into your lifestyle. This chapter offers guidance on best practices for using Tribulus, combining it with other supplements, and leveraging a balanced diet and healthy habits to optimize results.

Best Practices for Use

1. **Start with the Right Dosage**:
   - Begin with a **low dose** to gauge your body's response. Most supplements recommend **250–750 mg daily**, with higher doses often divided into two or three smaller servings.
   - If your goal is to support testosterone or libido, check for a product standardized for **40–60% saponins**, as these active compounds are associated with hormonal benefits.
2. **Follow a Schedule**:
   - Consistency is key. Take Tribulus at the same time(s) each day, preferably with meals, to enhance absorption and reduce the risk of digestive discomfort.

- Many users prefer a morning dose to align with natural hormonal rhythms or a split dose for sustained effects throughout the day.

3. **Cycle Its Use**:
    - To maintain effectiveness and minimize potential side effects, consider **cycling** Tribulus. A common approach is **4–6 weeks on, followed by 1–2 weeks off**.
    - Cycling prevents the body from adapting to the supplement, ensuring it remains effective over time.

4. **Monitor Your Body**:
    - Keep track of any changes in energy, mood, libido, or other symptoms. If you notice adverse effects like irritability or digestive issues, reduce the dosage or

discontinue use and consult a healthcare professional.

Combining with Other Supplements or Treatments

Tribulus Terrestris can be a powerful tool on its own, but it may also complement other supplements or treatments when used strategically.

1. **Pairing with Adaptogens**:
    - Combining Tribulus with adaptogens like **ashwagandha** or **rhodiola rosea** can help balance stress hormones and support overall vitality. While Tribulus targets testosterone and libido, adaptogens enhance resilience and energy levels.
2. **Supporting Joint and Muscle Health**:

- Athletes often pair Tribulus with supplements like **creatine** or **branched-chain amino acids (BCAAs)** to improve performance and recovery. The potential testosterone-boosting effects of Tribulus may enhance muscle growth when combined with these compounds.

3. **Boosting Cardiovascular Health**:
    - Tribulus's potential cardiovascular benefits make it a natural partner for omega-3 fatty acids or CoQ10, which are known for supporting heart health. This combination can be especially beneficial for individuals with a focus on endurance training or overall wellness.

4. **Complementing Sexual Health Regimens**:

- For libido or sexual health concerns, Tribulus can be paired with supplements like **maca root**, **L-arginine**, or **ginseng**, which also target sexual vitality and blood flow.

5. **Avoiding Negative Interactions**:
    - Always consult a healthcare professional before combining Tribulus with prescription medications or other supplements. For example, combining it with blood-thinning agents or certain hormonal therapies can pose risks.

Role in Diet and Lifestyle

Supplements like Tribulus Terrestris are most effective when integrated into a comprehensive approach to health, including diet, exercise, and lifestyle habits.

1. **Nutrient-Rich Diet**:
    - Enhance the benefits of Tribulus by maintaining a diet rich in whole foods. Focus on:
        - **Protein Sources**: Lean meats, fish, eggs, and plant-based proteins to support muscle repair and hormone production.
        - **Healthy Fats**: Nuts, seeds, avocado, and olive oil to provide essential building blocks for testosterone synthesis.
        - **Micronutrient Support**: Foods high in **zinc**, **magnesium**, and **vitamin D**, such as shellfish, pumpkin seeds,

and fortified foods, to further promote hormonal health.

2. **Stay Hydrated**:
   - Tribulus may have mild diuretic effects, so staying hydrated is crucial. Aim for at least **8–10 cups of water daily**, adjusting for activity levels and climate.

3. **Exercise Regularly**:
   - Physical activity is essential for maintaining optimal hormone levels. Combine Tribulus with:
     - **Strength Training**: Exercises like weightlifting boost testosterone production naturally and complement the herb's effects.
     - **Cardiovascular Activity**: Running, cycling, or swimming

supports cardiovascular health, an area where Tribulus has shown potential benefits.

4. **Manage Stress**:
    - Chronic stress elevates cortisol, which can suppress testosterone. Incorporate stress-reducing practices like **meditation, yoga**, or **deep breathing exercises** to enhance the effects of Tribulus.

5. **Get Quality Sleep**:
    - Hormones like testosterone are produced during deep sleep. Aim for **7–9 hours of restful sleep per night**, and establish a consistent bedtime routine to optimize recovery and hormone balance.

6. **Avoid Hormone-Disrupting Habits**:

- Minimize exposure to toxins, such as those in **processed foods**, **plastics**, and **alcohol**, which can disrupt endocrine function. A clean lifestyle amplifies the potential benefits of Tribulus.

Personalizing Your Routine

Every individual responds differently to supplements like Tribulus Terrestris. Factors such as age, activity level, and health status all play a role in determining the best approach.

- **For Athletes**: Incorporate Tribulus into a performance-focused regimen alongside a protein-rich diet and regular strength training.
- **For Libido and Sexual Health**: Pair Tribulus with stress-reducing techniques, intimate communication,

and supplements like L-arginine or maca root.
- **For Overall Wellness**: Combine Tribulus with adaptogens and a balanced lifestyle to support vitality and energy.

Tribulus Terrestris offers numerous benefits, but its effectiveness depends largely on how it's used. By following best practices, combining it thoughtfully with other supplements, and adopting a healthy lifestyle, you can maximize its potential while aligning it with your personal health goals. Whether you're seeking hormonal support, athletic performance, or general vitality, a well-rounded approach ensures lasting results and a sustainable routine.

CHAPTER 10:
Conclusion and Future Perspectives

Tribulus Terrestris has been celebrated for centuries, particularly for its reputed ability to enhance testosterone levels, boost libido, and support overall vitality. Whether you're seeking a natural way to improve athletic performance, manage hormonal health, or simply feel more energized, this remarkable plant offers a variety of potential benefits. However, like any supplement, it's important to approach its use thoughtfully and be aware of both its strengths and limitations. As the scientific community continues to explore its full potential, the future of Tribulus Terrestris supplementation remains promising but requires careful consideration.

Summary of Benefits and Challenges

Benefits:

1. **Hormonal Support**: The most well-known benefit of Tribulus is its ability to support **testosterone levels**, especially in individuals with mild deficiencies. This can enhance physical performance, muscle mass, and energy levels, making it a popular choice for athletes and those seeking to combat the effects of aging.
2. **Libido and Sexual Health**: Many users turn to Tribulus for its potential role in improving **libido** and addressing sexual dysfunction. While the evidence is still mixed, several studies suggest it can positively affect

sexual health by enhancing arousal and supporting healthy sexual function.

3. **Cardiovascular and General Wellness**:

   Beyond hormones and libido, Tribulus has shown promise in supporting **cardiovascular health**, reducing **inflammation**, and acting as an **antioxidant**. These benefits can contribute to overall vitality and improve the body's ability to manage stress and oxidative damage.

4. **Urinary and Reproductive Health**:

   Traditional uses of Tribulus include supporting **urinary health** and reproductive function, particularly for **men** dealing with **prostate** or **urinary tract issues**.

Challenges:

1. **Inconsistent Research Findings**: While many studies tout Tribulus as a powerful testosterone booster, others show minimal to no effect. This variability may stem from differences in **dosage**, **standardization of extracts**, or the **methodology** of individual studies. The lack of consensus makes it difficult to definitively declare Tribulus a miracle supplement for testosterone.
2. **Adulteration and Quality Control**: The supplement market can be rife with adulterated or poorly manufactured products. Some Tribulus supplements contain low levels of active compounds or may be mixed with fillers, reducing their overall effectiveness. It's crucial for consumers to identify high-quality products through certifications and transparency in labeling.

3. **Side Effects and Interactions**: Though generally regarded as safe, Tribulus can cause side effects in some users, including **gastrointestinal discomfort** or **mild irritability**. Additionally, potential interactions with medications or existing conditions—such as hormone-sensitive cancers—should be considered, making it essential to consult with a healthcare provider before use.

Emerging Research Areas

While Tribulus has a long history of use, the scientific exploration into its full potential is still ongoing. Here are a few emerging research areas that could shape the future of Tribulus supplementation:

1. **Mechanisms Behind Testosterone Boosting**:

Research into how Tribulus influences testosterone levels is still evolving. While some studies suggest that compounds like **protodioscin** and **saponins** may play a role, scientists are still uncovering the exact biochemical pathways involved. Future studies may provide more definitive answers and help tailor Tribulus supplements to specific needs.

2. **Impact on Women's Health**: Traditionally, Tribulus has been marketed primarily for men, but there's growing interest in its effects on **women's hormonal health**. Some studies indicate that Tribulus may help balance female hormones, improve **libido**, and even manage conditions like **PCOS** (polycystic ovary syndrome). Ongoing research could shed more light on its potential benefits for women.

3. **Tribulus and Mental Health**: There is some evidence that Tribulus may support **mental clarity** and **mood regulation** by balancing hormones related to stress and fatigue. Studies are starting to explore how Tribulus might play a role in reducing **anxiety** or **depression** related to hormonal imbalances. This is an exciting area of research that could expand the scope of Tribulus as an all-encompassing wellness supplement.

4. **Synergistic Effects with Other Herbs**:
   While Tribulus has been studied largely in isolation, researchers are beginning to investigate how it may work in synergy with other adaptogens or herbs. For example, pairing Tribulus with **ashwagandha, ginseng,** or **maca root** could lead to more potent

results, addressing multiple aspects of physical and mental well-being.

5. **Long-Term Safety and Efficacy**: Most Tribulus research focuses on short-term use, and there's limited data on its **long-term safety** and efficacy. Future studies examining the effects of prolonged use will be crucial in determining the sustainability of Tribulus supplementation and its potential risks when taken over extended periods.

Personalizing Supplementation for Optimal Results

While Tribulus Terrestris can be a valuable addition to many health routines, personalizing its use is key to achieving the best results. Here's how to tailor supplementation based on individual goals:

1. **Testosterone Support and Muscle Building**: If your primary goal is to boost testosterone for athletic performance or muscle growth, pair Tribulus with a consistent **strength training** program and a **protein-rich diet**. The optimal dosage may vary, but most athletes find that **500–750 mg** daily, in divided doses, works best. Combining Tribulus with **creatine** and **BCAAs** can further enhance muscle recovery and performance.

2. **Libido and Sexual Health**: For those using Tribulus to address **libido issues**, a lower dose (around **250–500 mg**) may be sufficient. Consider pairing Tribulus with **L-arginine** or **ginseng**, which improve blood flow and sexual function. Lifestyle factors such as reducing stress and improving sleep quality can also

amplify Tribulus's effects on sexual health.

3. **General Wellness**: If your goal is overall vitality and wellness, Tribulus can be a helpful addition to an adaptogenic stack that includes **ashwagandha** or **rhodiola rosea**. These herbs help balance the body's response to stress while supporting energy and endurance. Take Tribulus as part of a daily routine that includes a nutrient-dense diet and regular physical activity.

4. **Cycle and Monitor Progress**: For best results, consider **cycling** Tribulus and monitoring your progress. Take it for **4–6 weeks**, followed by a break, to prevent the body from adapting to its effects. Track changes in energy, mood, libido, or physical performance, and adjust the dosage or

combination of supplements as necessary.

Final Thoughts

Tribulus Terrestris holds a wealth of potential, but like any supplement, it works best when part of a well-rounded approach to health. Whether you're hoping to enhance testosterone levels, improve sexual health, or boost overall energy, Tribulus can be a valuable tool. The future of Tribulus supplementation looks promising, with emerging research offering new insights into its mechanisms and potential benefits. By personalizing your approach, remaining informed, and staying up-to-date with new findings, you can make the most of this time-honored herb.

www.ingramcontent.com/pod-product-compliance
Lightning Source LLC
Chambersburg PA
CBHW071412220526
45469CB00004B/1262